#Irefuse

TO STOP BEING ME

Alopecia Awareness Edition

of

CONFINEMENT CHRONICLES

Encouraging Testimonies Birthed Out

of the 2020 Pandemic

Stories Compiled by Angie BEE & Bartee
Productions

Edited by Zaundra George

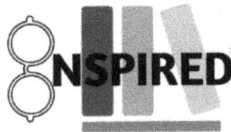

NSPIRED

Reading for the Whole Person

INSPIRED published by
Ladero Press LLC
2763 Lighthouse Cove Road
Orange City, Florida 32763

First Ladero Press Printing, August 2022

#Irefuse to Stop Being Me
Alopecia Awareness Edition of
Confinement Chronicles:
Encouraging Testimonies Birthed Out of the 2020 Pandemic

Contains previously printed content.

ISBN: 978-1-946981-84-4 Paperback /
978-1-946981-85-1 EPUB /
978-1-946981-86-8 KPF

Printed in the United States of America
Set in Quattrocento Sans, and Objectivity ExtBd.
Cover Designed by SheerGenius

Library of Congress information available upon request.
www.laderopress.com

TABLE OF CONTENTS

#Irefuse

TO STOP BEING ME

VOLUME IX

Confinement Chronicles
A fundraiser for
Baldie
THE MOVEMENT
*Improving our Mental Health
by sharing stories of hair loss & survival*

#Irefuse to stop being ME!
2 Corinthians 1:3-4
An inspirational audiobook compilation series inspired by the 2020 Pandemic. Produced by
Bee Productions
Ministry, media and more

INTRODUCTION

Why a book about Alopecia? Why not? I've got it, she's got it, he's got it, they've got it; there are a whole lot of people dealing with this autoimmune disease, and several of them shared their stories in this book.

When I first realized my hair was thinning, I didn't really panic because my mother had thinning hair; but when the bald patches appeared, I panicked. You see, I grew up in a household where my dad *lovvvvvvveddddddd* long, thick, luxurious hair. He would fuss at my baby sister if she thought about cutting her hair. He thought women were beautiful with long, thick, luxurious hair, and I could not see myself approaching my dad with a bald head.

So, what did I do? I put on a wig, and I proceeded to hide under that wig for decades. Thank God for hot flashes! They helped me begin to snatch this wig off my head, and once the wig was off, I started to look at myself differently. I always thought I was kinda cute with a round head . . . I thought. Then, I met my husband Bartee: on our first date, I told him, "You need to understand, this wig comes off," and I took it off, thinking it would scare him away (LOL). Instead, he smiled and looked at me . . . the rest of the story is written in our first book entitled *In the Beginning: There Was God, Me & You.*

As most autoimmune disorders go, alopecia is on the mild side: it doesn't force us to go into the hospital, and we don't have to take medication to treat it, unlike other autoimmune disorders. There is no cure for our disease because it's considered cosmetic. A bald man is considered **sexy**; a bald child is considered **weird** and is oftentimes bullied; but a bald woman has been called butch, rebellious, unchristian, ugly, and so forth.

Over the years serving as an ambassador for alopecia, I have learned that there are many types. Each person has struggled with their individual diagnosis in their own way; some have been outed, others have been embarrassed, but we all have a similar journey where we had to come to grips with the cards we were dealt.

In this book, the stories originally printed in *Confinement Chronicles: Encouraging Testimonies Birthed Out of the 2020 Pandemic*, you will read stories from several "Alopecians" like myself and a few supporters, as well.

We thank you for reading. We thank you for listening and we thank you for sharing. Be safe and BEE Blessed!

Evangelist Angie BEE

During a recent radio interview, my husband Bartee and I were asked about the Bold Beautiful & Bald Beauty Bazaar. This Alopecia Awareness weekend is an annual fundraiser that takes place in Daytona Beach, Florida, each September, during Alopecia Awareness month. As I shared my hair loss story with the audience, and my husband contributed his thoughts, a beautiful revelation of God's goodness and direction began to unfold before my very eyes. If I had not begun to lose my hair more than twenty years ago, I would not have been able to encourage another person on their journey of hair loss and re-discovery. I am grateful for that revelation!

Now, as we present these stories of hair loss for our Alopecia Awareness audiobook volume, I see how that re-discovery is present in each of our authors. The beginning of our stories may be similar:

- we started losing our hair
- someone noticed and told us that we were losing our hair
- we covered our hair loss in a variety of ways

But now we are each serving a greater calling by helping others in our own special way!

From hair loss to a greater purpose! LOOK AT GOD!

We have arrived at Volume IX and, although it may have been delivered to listeners a bit out of order (Volume VII debuted on September 1, 2020) these words that you are about to experience are WELL WORTH THE WAIT!

And now, for our first contribution...

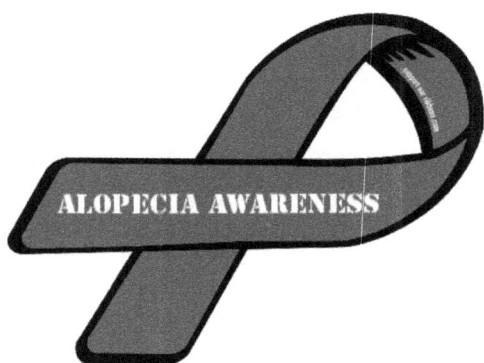
ALOPECIA AWARENESS

SUMMARY OF MY HAIR STORY

By Michelle Walters - Johnson

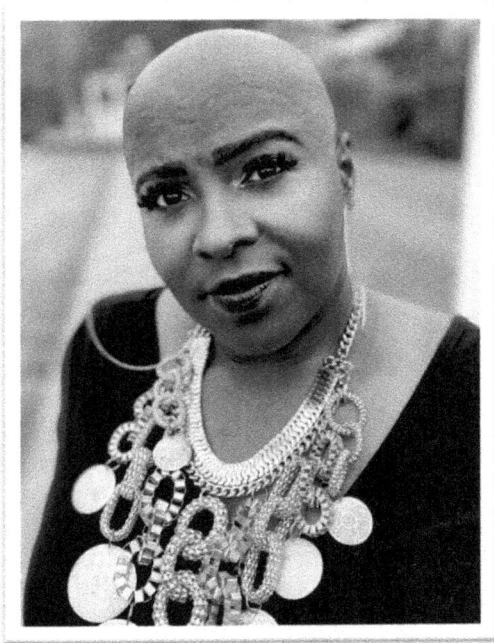

I n my experience, my hair loss began at the age of twenty-eight. I was living life, minding my business, and one day my mother came to visit from out of town, and one of her first comments to me was about how thin my hair was. Up until this point, I actually never noticed the hair thinning. But once I really took a look, I came to the realization that my hair was not as thick as it used to be. I have had a love/hate relationship with my hair and with this whole process since then.

My love affair with wigs started after the birth of my daughter fifteen years ago. After her birth, my hair thinned out considerably. I became a professional at learning how to blend my hair with the partial wig. I typically wore them about shoulder length or in a bob so that they were very natural looking. I don't think too many people realized it wasn't my hair. Wigs gave me that extra boost of confidence to try things that I had always wanted to do, but was afraid to, like modeling. But that's a story for another day.

Losing one's hair has a great psychological impact. For many women, hair loss can happen so fast, not giving them enough time to adjust. This can cause some to go into a deep depression. Add to that the fact that they may also be going through medical issues, extreme stress, or some other life impacting drama.

I will never forget the time when I was at a hairdresser appointment with my niece Tiara. We were getting ready to try a treatment, and she prayed over me. That moment is still etched in my head. She prayed that my hair loss would not affect my self-esteem; and I will honestly say from that time forward, I have not psychologically struggled with my hair loss.

Although I have not let Alopecia damage my self-esteem, there are plenty of women that do. This phenomenon gives a new charge to my business, instead of focusing on only creating wigs, I focus on helping women with alopecia feel better about themselves. I have been privileged to influence them to embrace their natural beauty and feel proud about showing their beautiful bald heads; and then if they desire, finding the right wig or wigs that further enhance their natural beauty. By coming forward with my truth, I believe that I have found my profound purpose.

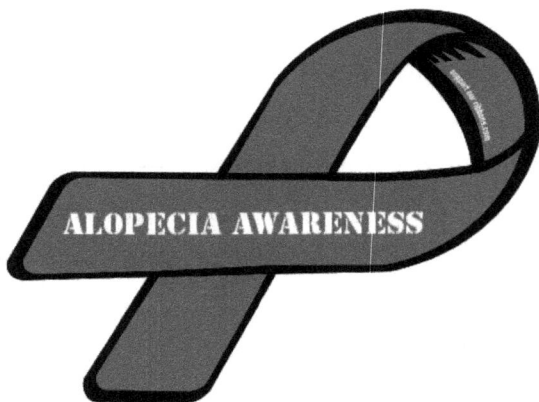

THE ADVENTURES OF A BALDIE....

By Lorna Mastin

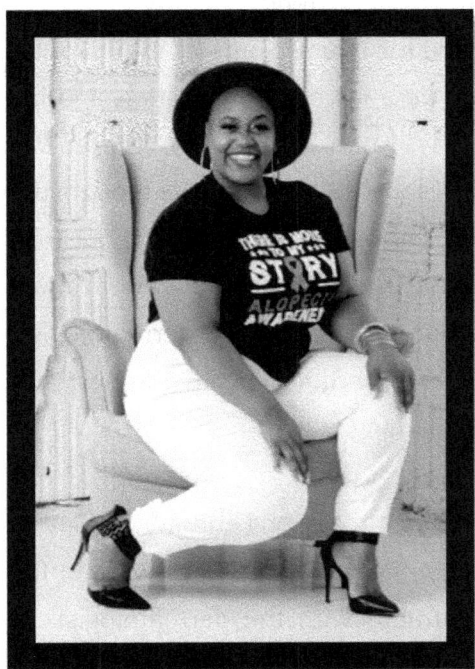

G rowing up in Southfield, Michigan, one of my fondest moments was getting my hair done. I had a very nice, soft texture of hair with great length. I was like my mom's personalized Barbie doll. Every hairstyle she wanted to try, she did it on me. I wasn't tender-headed, and I could sit there for hours. Some of my favorite hair styles were latch hook, twisties, and braids. One day, I noticed this tiny little bald spot. When I showed my mom, we thought maybe one of the braids had pulled it out from its tightness. Anywho, we decided to make an appointment for the dermatologist to examine everything, but we honestly didn't think anything of it.

One very cold day on February, the 14th to be exact, in the year of 2002, I went in for my appointment with the dermatologist. I was excited because I was able to get out of school early, but at the same time, attempting to be focused, because we had a volleyball game that day at 4 PM. (I did not play when it came to athletics; I'm very competitive.) So, my mom and I arrived, sat down, and in came the doctor. He examined my head and casually said, "Yeah ... looks like you have Alopecia." I had never heard of it, never knew anyone with it, and could not tell you where it came from. They said it could be hereditary or it could be triggered by stress. I was a little stressed as a teenager, but isn't everybody? So, I thought.

My mom asked about treatment, and it was then that the doctor shared the bitter reality that there was no cure, but we could "try" a few things. (I was thinking, *I know they don't think I'm going to be a guinea pig.*) So, they told us about these cortisone injections that work for some people, and that we could try it. I cried my eyes out asking for another option because I had a game that day, and I didn't think I could handle getting shots in my head and playing. They decided to give me some steroids that I could only take for a month because if I took too many, they could cause kidney failure. So, essentially I had thirty days to prepare my mind for the injections.

When I went back the following Monday, the injections began. Hair would grow in one spot then fall out again. We played this cat and mouse game for four years. Each month I'd go, and I would get anywhere from one hundred to one hundred twenty-six (100-126) injections in my head at a time. OOOoouch! In my senior year of high school, we tried one more thing. I was sent to a specialist, and we tried a light box treatment which ended up looking just like a tanning booth. The idea was that the UV light would stimulate the growth on my head. Well, after a year of that, the end result was actually little to no hair growth, and it tanned the rest of my face. So, my face ended up being darker than the rest of my body. At that point, I had had it! I was over the treatments because nothing was completely successful. Sometimes, I was able to cover up the areas where my hair fell out, and other times I wasn't, and had to wear wigs. Now, these wigs are not what the lace fronts look like today! They were the ones your great-grandmother wore that slid to the right or the left if you turned your head too quickly! An absolute disaster! I remember my ponytail clip falling off while trying to steal second base during a softball game. Or, the time my wig came off while playing volleyball. Or, it sliding alllll the way to the right during a meet as I threw the shot out in disgust! Not to mention all of this happening during high school, where absolutely everything matters. (But not really.)

I managed to make it through high school and decided for all treatments to come to an end. At fourteen, I knew God had a purpose for me experiencing this, but just wasn't sure what it was. Years had gone by, and I still hadn't met anyone with this same condition or that even looked like me and had alopecia. As time progressed, my hair started to grow back. It got really long, too. I was just waiting on my edges to come in. I had gotten married, had a great sew-in, and I thought I was in the clear. Unless you were blood family or really close friends, many still didn't know I suffered from Alopecia, but it didn't bother me as much because I could wear sew-ins to cover it up.

Welp, in 2015, I got pregnant with my son, and of course my hair grew like crazy, but when he came out in 2016, so did ALLLLLLL of my hair. This was tough. I was trying to hold onto the little I did have. I felt bad for my now ex-husband because he liked hair—long hair—and n order to give him that, I'd have to not be my natural self. Wearing or getting a sew-in is one thing, but having to wear a COMPLETE wig was another. By the grace of

God, I didn't really struggle with self-esteem due to this, because my mother constantly made sure we all knew we were loved and extraordinarily awesome, but I did.

In 2019, a series of events took place leading to a change in my relationship status, requiring me to do an overall rebuild. I felt that in this transitioning season as I began to rebuild certain parts of my life, everybody was going to have to get used to seeing me bald. I did a photoshoot with all my naturalness and posted it on social media January 1, 2020. I wasn't looking for approval, likes, shares, comments, support, or any of that! I just wanted people to know moving forward, that they were gonna get this bald head, and they needed to start accepting that like "Now!" LOL. Well, the response was astronomical. With thousands of likes, shares, and comments, I was blown away. Many encouraged me to not wear wigs and just be my natural self. As the days went on, I began to fall in love and be super comfortable with myself. The last time I wore a wig was when the Pandemic hit in March 2020.

I will be honest, I didn't know how dating would be, but to my surprise, men like bald women. LOL. Like A LOT of men. This journey of self-discovery has been exceptional. I've made it my mission to find and connect with women all over the world that have Alopecia and continue to educate the community on this auto-immune disease, and be a support to those who are struggling on their journey. I never thought the one area of my life that I was embarrassed, ashamed, and modified about would be the one thing that many love and appreciate about me. I guess it was God's plan all along!

Lorna Mastin

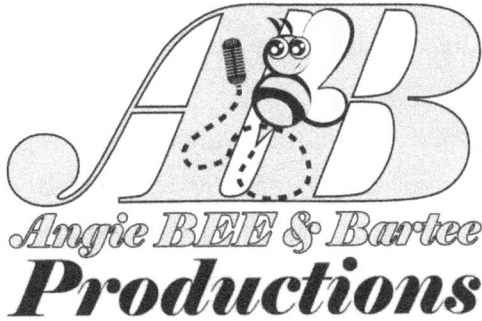

Angie BEE & Bartee
Productions

From the beginning, we knew this volume would spread Alopecia Awareness and encourage others that are facing hair loss. We also knew that we wanted to help raise funds for a non-profit organization by releasing this audiobook. The Lord heard our cry and pointed us in the direction of The Baldie Movement! With over nine thousand followers (9,000) on Facebook alone, this social media inspiration is a powerhouse! The Baldie Movement and its founder "Nellie Nell" truly deserve our support!

A portion of the proceeds raised by Angie BEE Productions on the audiobook volume will be donated to The Baldie Movement.

This next new author truly labored over her contribution; she really just struggled as to how to get her story from her head onto paper. Our team understood completely, so we invited her to submit her story by video. Once received, our expert transcriptionist "Sonya Bee" took Shay's words from the video and added them to paper. Now, you will hear her story, in her own voice!

SLAY AS YOU ARE
By Shay

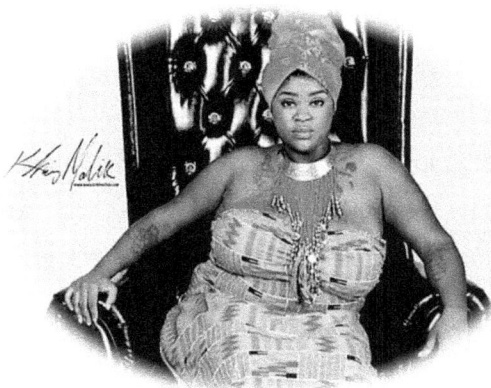

Hello, my name is Shay, and I am currently a hair stylist in Sacramento, California. I wanted to briefly share a little bit about my hair-loss journey. Unfortunately, you can't see it right now, but I lost my edges like most women. My journey of hair loss started when I was in high school – probably as early as middle school. Back in time, I received a perm at a very young age probably five, if not six, but I remember being young, and that started a process of me getting older and believing that I needed to perm my hair in order for it to be straight – not realizing that I was removing the natural coil of my hair. With that, I used to wear very tight braids, very tight singles. Literally, I had the motto, "If it wasn't tight, it wasn't right." Then eventually, I was introduced to hair-bonding glue "black glue", as we all know, for bonding tracks. As time went by, my not properly caring for it, my not properly being taught how to remove it, caused me to lose my edges and things.

I decided to want to be a hair stylist because as I got older and started to learn and study my craft, I realized there were so many women that I've connected with that suffer from the same condition that I have and who have lost confidence in this process. I believe that doing hair has given me the ability to connect with many different women on many different levels and has helped me to build a certain level of confidence within myself to be able to connect and share my own story of how I lost my edges and how I lost a lot of self-esteem behind it.

My goal, as I get deeper into my business, I will be launching a hair line the beginning of next year that's called, *Slay As You Are*. Eventually, I hope to be able to educate a lot of women on the self-esteem part of having hair loss. Even though my hair is done right now because I am a hair stylist, I have many times gone live on social media and things of that nature in my natural to let other women know, "Hey, you're not alone. Hey, that doesn't make you a bad person." Just back in time, we were not educated on certain things which resulted in losing hair. Eventually, I want to make wigs for women who have suffered from hair loss whether it be cancer, whether it be Alopecia, or all the other things that make women lose their hair. I want to be able to connect with them and make wigs and offer my services because I do believe when you have your hair done, it gives you the confidence you need.

I didn't realize that not only are young girls are suffering from it, but many adult women. I didn't realize that until I really started getting into my craft of doing hair; I learned a lot about women. Men suffer from it, but I am a woman, so I will address the womanly issue of confidence. I did not realize how many people and clients whose hair I have done were so ashamed to show who they were. Many times, my clients, who really know me, know that I'm quick to pull off their wigs if it's loose, and I can take it off to show them, "Hey, you're still beautiful; you're not your hair."

So, in saying that, I hope that my being able to share a little bit of myself and my journey will help other women to accept who they are, and if not, reach out to me and we can connect and network. We need it.

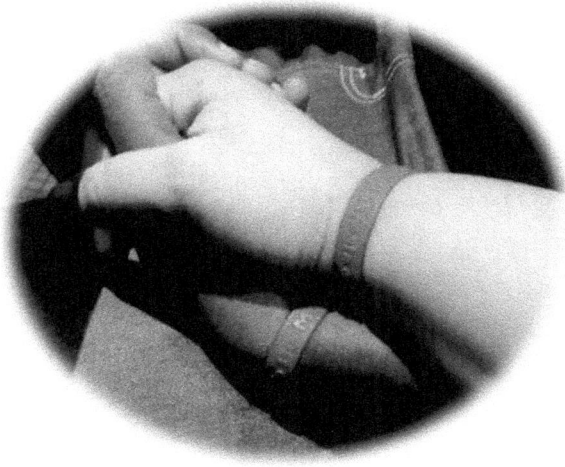

NO BAD HAIR DAYS
By Uniqua Leak

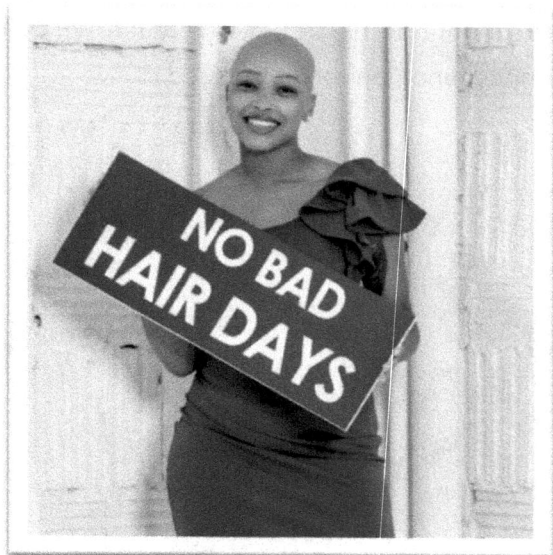

I am Uniqua Leak from Detroit, Michigan, and I have been living with Alopecia for twenty-three years. I was six years old when round-like patches of my hair began to come out. At this time, I really did not understand what was happening, and this did not immediately have an effect on me. I still had a good length of hair: it was thick, curly, and my hair stylist was able to cover the bald spots with various different styles. My grandmother wanted to find out the cause for my hair loss. I went to a number of dermatologists and cosmetologists. After being diagnosed with Alopecia Areata, I was told that the onset of my alopecia was caused from stress or trauma.

I began exploring different treatments. There was a topical cream which is a cream I applied twice daily to the bald areas on my scalp. There was an electric scalp stimulator tool for natural hair growth. None of these treatments seemed to help. Hair would grow in areas where it once was bald, but I would lose hair in other spots on my head. I got older, kids got meaner, treatments got higher in cost, and my hair began to come out faster. It was suggested that I try a more invasive treatment, known as Corticosteroid Injections. As a grade-school child I was unwilling to undergo such an invasive procedure because this involved injections on my scalp.

After having my second child in 2010, my hair rapidly began to shed. There were only two spots on opposite sides of my head where I still had hair. I was nineteen years old, and I had seen dozens of dermatologists. I was angry that treatments did not help in the past, so I decided to allow my child's father to help me shave the hair that was left on my head. I showered, combed my hair, and braided it into two different braids. We stood in the mirror of the bathroom, and as I began to cry, he shaved one braid off, and I lost all control of my emotions. I didn't let him shave the last braid. I kicked him out of the bathroom while screaming and crying. After what seemed to be hours, but more like thirty-to-forty-five minutes, I looked into the mirror and cut off the last braid. I wanted to hold on to the last braid. I found a small gold empty jewelry box. I placed both braids into the box to keep forever. This chapter is called "Shit Just Got Real."

I had to come up with a plan. I had no hair on my head for the first time in my life! What was I going to do? WIGS! I did not wear wigs or weaves when I had hair. This chapter I call, "My Frenemy." You know? You do not really like her, but you deal with her. It was a love-hate relationship. My aunt suggested I rock the bald look. When others would suggest this, it would make me angry, and I would tell them, "If you think it looks good, then shave your head and you rock it." The chemicals used in weaves and wigs did not agree with my skin. My face would break out. I tried wearing a lace front wig which had to be applied with hair glue and tape. Morgan (my first wig) was a 14-inch body wave curl. I wore her for a few months. Getting her reapplied became costly. I decided to learn to make my own wigs; I turned to You Tube. As time went on, and with a lot of practice, I got really good at this process. I grew comfortable with wearing wigs. I always wore only one style, shoulder length, blondish brown and curly. Same style I had before losing all my hair.

If not having hair on my head wasn't stressful and depressing enough, I began to lose my eyebrows. This chapter I call, "Seriously, Was the Hair on my Head Not Enough?" I honestly did not think this would be so hard on me. I was a pretty good artist. I loved to paint and draw, so I thought I could draw some eyebrows. LOL. I was so wrong. I could never draw two that looked the same. I was not a fan of having to draw on eyebrows several times a day.

Friends and family would ask all the time, "Why don't you wear your real hair anymore?" This would bother me. I did not want to explain that I have an autoimmune disease and my body is attacking my hair follicles. In 2017, I did just that! I decided to take to Facebook to reach a larger number of people. I posted two photos. One with my homemade curly wig and the other of myself with no wig. People that I have known most of my life commented in surprise, not knowing that I had been battling with hair loss. Others applauded my courage to share something so personal with the world. I cried while reading every comment. I felt like I had freed myself from this box that was sealed for so long.

As a result of my Facebook post, I was introduced to microblading, a tattooing technique that was a game changer for my "Slay, Sis" chapter. Microblading helped with my confidence greatly. I no longer needed to spend hours drawing brows on my face. The tattoos looked so natural, and I was happy.

The following year in 2018, I learned how to do headwraps. That April, I decided to put all of the weaves, glue, wigs, and head caps in the trash. I was done wearing fake hair. My twenty-seventh birthday was coming up; I had a trip planned to soak up the sun on the beach of Mexico. I arrived wearing a head scarf. Once it was time to hit the beach, the headwrap came off. I felt free! There was no one there that I knew. I told myself, "These people do not know you, so who cares if they stare!" There was a lot of staring, and I did not care. This is "Free."

The biggest test I had ahead of me was returning home to face my peers. My confidence grew. I went everywhere rocking my bald head. I received compliments all the time.

These last two years, I have chosen to love myself fearlessly. I am never looking back!

MY ALOPECIA SHORT STORY ...

By Tamara R. Flake

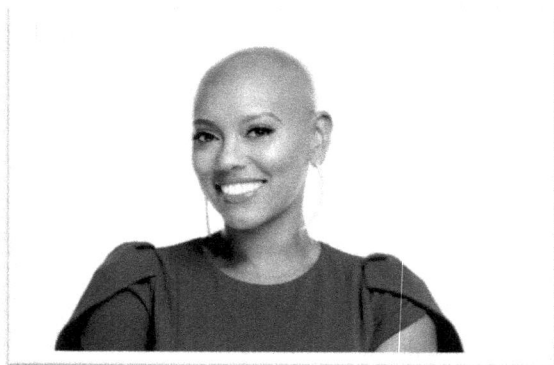

A t the age of six, I began to develop dime- and quarter-sized bald spots on my head, and my parents had no idea why. See, I thought it was because I cut my hair one time in first grade with the not-so-sharp scissors they gave us in school. My parents scheduled me an appointment with the dermatologist, and that is when I was diagnosed with Alopecia Areata. Between the ages of six to twenty-nine, alopecia was a constant thought and struggle for me. I was always thinking of a way to hide my baldness under wigs, hats, headwraps and weaves. Alopecia Areata makes it difficult to wear your own hair in many stages because you experience random bald patches of all sizes throughout your head. So, I was obsessed with keeping my secret, even though it was blatantly obvious that the hair on my head was not mine, and I was clearly wearing a wig or weave. As I grew older, I was more conscious of making the wigs and weaves look more natural which was extremely expensive, but worth it to me, to avoid the stares, embarrassment, and questions.

As a kid in the 80s, it was tough wearing wigs because I did not have all the wig options that are available for kids today. I wanted so badly to wear cornrows, box braids, and ponytails, but my only options were wigs from the beauty supply store made for adult women. I was afraid to participate in sports, water activities, and anything physical for fear of my wig coming off. The only thing securing the wig to my head was the stretch band inside of it, which was not very secure at all. There was no glue or tape available back then to secure the hair to my head, and I lived in constant fear of being exposed if the wig came off, or if God forbid, someone snatched it off my head, which did happen when I was thirteen.

Fast forward to adulthood . . . I thought not having hair would hold me back from advancing professionally. It was still a process to stop wearing my wigs to work even though I had been bald in my personal life for three years before. It was liberating to stop hiding at work because it was the final step to fully embracing my truth. I had been building up to it for months. Setting dates and breaking them. For example, one time, I said my New Year's resolution would be to go to work without my wig on. THAT DIDN'T HAPPEN!! I realized I was still holding on to fear and shame of who I really was. So, I began to educate my staff, business partners, and clients about alopecia and tell them my story. I would show them pictures of me without hair to gauge their reactions. I was doing all of this to build up my courage to come to work without the hair and to gain their support whenever I decided to do so.

Support is important to have through this process. I have always had a strong support system with my family. So, in my mind, I needed the support of my work family to get through this next phase in my journey. Finally, on April 23, 2012 (thanks for the memory Facebook), I DID IT! I went to work without my hair. I made sure my makeup was on point, and I was dressed really cute and professionally with the perfect accessories. I walked in that building with my head high and an attitude that said, "I am strong. I am Bold. I am courageous. I am beautiful. I AM UNAPOLOGETICALLY ME!"

Alopecia was once something that I was ashamed of having; however, when I felt that way, it was because I wanted to be like everyone else. That time, between ages six and twenty-nine, was a major growth phase for me. It took time for me to learn who Tamara truly is. It was a process ... a journey that I needed to experience to arrive at my authenticity. Now, I LOVE that Alopecia makes me different! I stand out, and I am not like anyone else. I have a story to share to empower and encourage someone who needs to hear it. Alopecia has freed me to be my true authentic self, and that is a woman I can be proud of! I do not hide; I am not afraid; I live life to the fullest and embrace every experience without fear of being exposed and embarrassed. I took my power back. I am uniquely me, and I would not trade me for anyone else in the world!

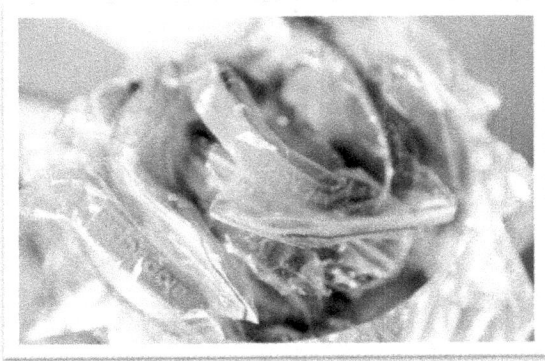

Photo by Jhonn de la Puente
www.facebook.com/jdlpphotography

THE STORY OF BOLD AND BALDNESS

By Raquel Johnson

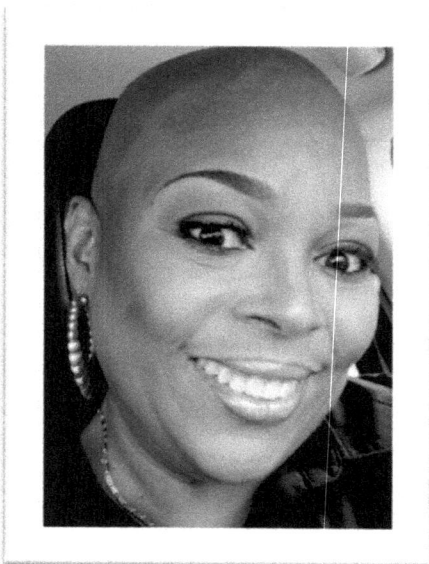

I grew up in Detroit, Michigan, where I come from a family of cosmetologists and barbers. My dad was a licensed Cosmetologist/Barber whose primary focus was healthy hair. He owned his own barber shop on Harper and Dickerson named Exodus. Having three children, two girls and boy, and my mother, who was the wife, it was my dad's responsibility to provide haircare for his family.

My hair was long, super thick, and hard to manage. I can remember my dad performing electro treatments, specialized conditions, and constant brushing, along with massaging my scalp and my mother's, as well. He took great pride in growing my hair until his untimely passing at the age of thirty-three. I was only ten years old when my father went to sleep and died as a result of a brain aneurysm. My hair continued to grow and grow. The thickness and texture were so strong. I was always told by beauticians that I had a good head of hair to work with.

I am fifty years old today. In my thirties, which was in the 2000s, I noticed that my hair began to thin out in such a way that I was forced to wear braids or hair weave with the hopes of covering up those thin spots. Well, the covering up only lasted for so long. My hair began to come out around the frontal part of my head and in the center. I was about thirty-six years old when I made my first appointment to see a dermatologist. It was then I was told by my doctor that I had alopecia. My doctor began to tell me about treatments, which were the injections that I began to hate so badly. After a few years of constantly going to see the dermatologist and getting those awful painful injections that did not help my situation, I began to become more frustrated day by day. At that point in my life, I began to buy human hair and get full hair weaves that were sewed onto French braids. Ohhh! I thought this was the lifetime fix. Something I could afford and looked nice, and no one knew about the severe thinning underneath. After four-to-five years of wearing weaves/sew-ins, my hair began to fall out all around the front and in the top. I was no longer able to get a regular weave. It was that day when I began to follow this young man named Richard Anthony on Facebook who was in Atlanta, Georgia.

Richard Anthony is a stylist in Atlanta who specializes in making hair units for women who suffer from alopecia. His technique is unbelievable. My mother would help finance my trips to Atlanta, Georgia, to get custom wigs made by the one and only Richard Anthony B.K.A. Prince Charming. These wigs would cost me anywhere between four hundred to seven hundred dollars. They were handmade and would last for a few years. I would wear what is called frontals or 360s. These wigs came with customized hair lines and parts throughout the wig that looks like your regular scalp. The wigs were awfully expensive until I found a young lady in Detroit named Marlene Brooks who was able to customize wigs and sew-ins, as well. I rocked those wigs and frontal sew-ins for years without many people knowing about my hair condition. At this point in my life, I was not able to grow hair anywhere but around the side. My hair was completely gone in the top and all around the front.

In 2016 to 2020, a series of events began to happen. In 2016, I lost my first cousin Tamela Wolfe to brain cancer. She was only forty-seven years old. I was devastated, and it sent me into depression. On February 10, 2018, my beautiful mother suffered a massive stroke right before my eyes as she was showing me how to use my snow blower. My mother was my everything. My mother held on at the hospital for seven days and transitioned on February 17. I was broken and did not know how to move forward without her. I did the work and attended grief counseling, and I also participated in a support grief support. On March 25, 2020, during COVID-19, I lost my only brother whose name was Orlando Johnson. He suffered a massive heart attack; they think he may have also had COVID-19. The medical examiner stated that he had pneumonia, but they did not give him a test for COVID-19 because he expired in the ambulance. My brother's death sent me back into depression.

My sister and I laid my brother away as we knew my mom would want us to. It was at this point where I had just had enough! I never wanted to disclose the fact that I had alopecia. My brother's daughter was angry with me and my sister after my brother passed. My family has always been close and stuck together with each other. My niece threatened to disclose my baldhead on Facebook. I panicked; I did not know what to do. I was so angry because I did not want anyone to know that I suffered from alopecia. A few days later, I made the decision to shave my hair off and acknowledge that I am an alopecia survivor. My reveal on Facebook was overwhelming. I received over five hundred-plus positive posts. I thank God for allowing me to reveal my bald head and tell my story. My name is Raquel Johnson, and I have survived Alopecia.

THERE'S BEAUTY IN YOUR FLAWS

A Poem by Shay

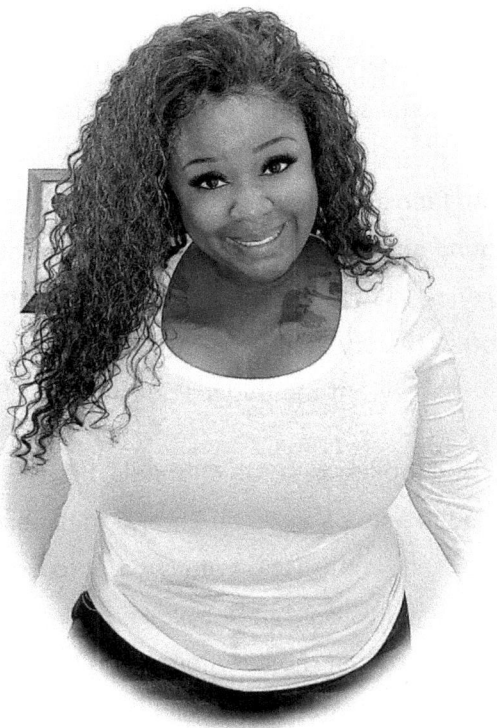

What does it mean to be beautiful?
You see, that's now the answer I seek,
because growing up I always thought beauty
was considered skin deep.
Way past what the eyes could see yet, you
see I'm standing here all dolled up and
pretty, still seeking the definition of beauty.
I got all my eyelashes on, I even painted on
my face an' dang; can you believe I even
found something to slim down my waist!?
Trying to fit into what society sees as the
perfect beauty; and can you believe it I even
want that bigger booty?

So I looked at some channels, flipped
through some shows on TV and then asked
myself "Is this who I really want to be?
Because this is what people see as reality,
no, no, that most definitely ain't me.
But just sit back and relax as I flip to the next
chapter and show you a different form of
me. Let's just called this next chapter:

"The Purist Form of the real and natural me".

Well, here I am just as natural as can be
"The Realist Form of *Natural ol' Me*".
So tell me, do I now fit in; Now that I've
uncovered the real me? Now that I've
showed you as natural as I can be? No
edges, no makeup, my lace front now gone,
but don't make me feel like I did some kind
of wrong!
You see it's time we learn to realize that this
too is beauty. It's just what you would call a
Real Natural Beauty, so let's not throw shade
on another sister's flaws because, truth be
told, we all got some kind of flaw. Some
choose to hide it, while others stand tall, but
sista... I'm here to help u to learn to embrace
them all!

So love yourself and don't be afraid to be
free and if and when you do always
remember this is the natural ol' me.

HOW CAN I NOT LIKE A BOLD, BEAUTIFUL AND BALD WOMAN?

By Bartee

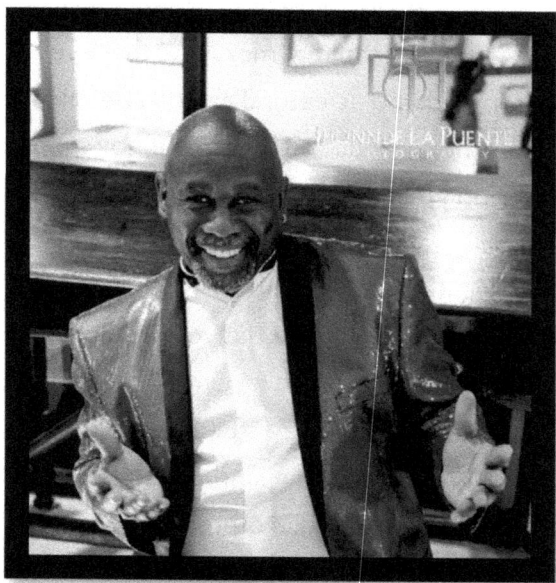

Y ou know, after listening to some jazz music, I told Angela that she had some pretty lips. I asked her if I could kiss her. Her response was (I really don't remember what she said), but anyway, we kissed! After sitting down and talking with each other about matters of the heart, Angela explained to me that she had a mental illness, and we talked about that for a while. Then, she took off her wig and explained to me that she had Alopecia (although I didn't know what that meant at the time).

First of all, let me state that she looked like a "China Baby" with her smooth, clear, shiny bald head. I kinda smiled because I didn't see any knots or bumps or hills to climb (LOL!), if you know what I mean. So, with that, I was good!

Now, it would have been another story if her head wasn't as smooth and shaped like a China Baby! And you know, knowing me, I would have told her, "Hey, you know, maybe you need to keep that wig on and maybe cut it down a little bit" because her wig was kinda long and thick, and I knew it was a wig in the first place (LOL).

Everyone is not as fortunate to have a nice round scalp for a bald head, so one must have enough confidence in themselves to wear that type of look – that Baldie Look! So, to say what I need to say, "Be Bold, Beautiful and Bald!"

MY STORY
By Evangelist Angie BEE

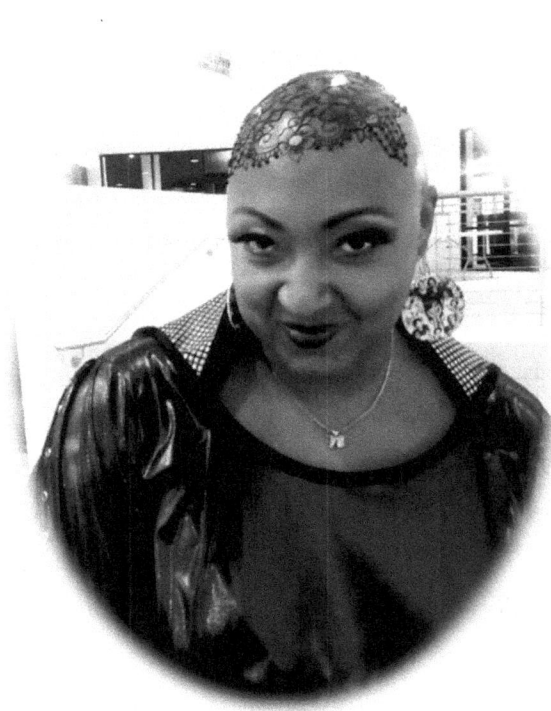

This photo was taken at the 2019 Bold Beautiful & Bald Beauty Bazaar in Daytona Beach, Florida.

My gown and cape were created by Senia Soto of Jarix Designs. My earrings were created by Arlene Hall-Scarlett, CEO of Novyedesigns.

Tiffany Tyson Green of Sophisticated Tips adorned me with my eyelashes, and my henna "crown" came from one of our event vendors.

My contribution was originally printed in the September 2020 issue of *Triumphant Magazine*. This inspirational publication has featured our *Confinement Chronicles* authors each month since we first launched our audiobook series. Search for *Triumphant Magazine* on Facebook and tell publisher Theresa Jordan that we are so grateful for her support. This is My Story.

September is Alopecia Awareness Month, so if you begin to see a lot of royal blue images everywhere, that is because men, women, and children just like me are celebrating and sharing what we live with as Alopecians!

Although I preach, speak, lead workshops, and appear on Facebook LIVE each week with my bald head glistening, people still ask me, *"Angie BEE, why are you bald? Don't you want to try a wig to cover your head? Are you sick? Are you having treatments? Would you like to try this and that to make your hair grow?"*

So, let's have a conversation. According to the National Alopecia Areata Foundation at www.NAAF.org, *"Alopecia areata is a common autoimmune skin disease, causing hair loss on the scalp, face and sometimes on other areas of the body. In fact, it affects as many as 6.8 million people in the U.S. with a lifetime risk of 2.1%"*. I unknowingly started showing signs of this disease in 1995. My then-hairdresser offered to glue in a weave to cover the bald patches that she saw. I didn't see them, and she wanted to try something new, so I agreed to it! Not long after that, my daughters and I were in a head-on collision with an 18-wheel semi-tractor, pulling a trailer. During my recovery, as my mother was combing my hair, she immediately recognized my bald spaces.

"Angie, you have Alopecia. My dermatologist diagnosed me with a form of it too," my mother told me.

In 2017, Donna Gray-Banks encouraged me and Bartee to launch an annual event that allows those with alopecia to gather together in a social and informative session to learn and network. The Bold Beautiful & Bald Beauty Bazaar debuted as a one-day shopping and fashion event in Daytona Beach, Volusia County, Florida. Each year the event has doubled in size, and in 2018, we even added a Weekend Beachside Retreat! Fashion show models, sponsors, guests, and friends gather at a designated host resort and enjoy evening s'mores, photo shoots, a dinner boat cruise, workshops, and fellowship. Last year, we learned how to apply magnetic eyelashes (when you have no eyelashes or eyebrows, this is an important class to have). The year prior, we learned about financing, marriage and relationship tips from Author Kayl May (Atlanta), and "Stan the State Farm Insurance Man" Stan Harrison of New Smyrna Beach, Florida.

There were even two lovebirds that attended our 2018 weekend retreat relationship workshop, and now they are married! One of them has alopecia and the other one doesn't care. They see each other for who they are and how God brought them together! They are BLESSED!

The next time you see a bald person, don't stare, don't frown, don't whisper, or turn away. Give us a BIG smile and a THUMBS UP because you don't know the journey it took for us to snatch off those wigs and flaunt our beautiful bald heads!

Learn more about our annual Alopecia Awareness weekend event at www.BoldBeautifulAndBald.com and follow us at www.Facebook.com/BoldBeautifulAndBald BeautyBazaar

Sometimes, an author needs to speak his/her words using a video camera or an audio recorder. Afterwards, a true talent like SONYA BENNETT can transcribe those words, and even include the correct punctuation, all in print. A very special thank you to Sonya for transcribing the video submitted to this project. Thank you for helping me to capture and include those words in this issue of *Confinement Chronicles*.

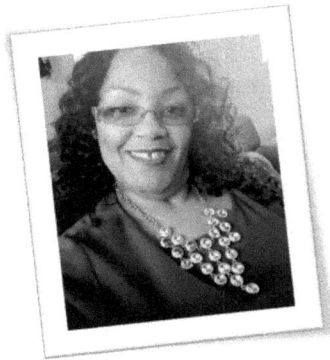

Sonya Bennett, Author / Narrator and Professional Transcriptionist with Angie BEE Productions

This concludes *Confinement Chronicle*s and the #IrefuseToStopBeingMe volume, which serves as a fundraiser for The Baldie Movement. A portion of the proceeds from this project were donated to this 501C3-non-profit organization, and we invite YOU to make a donation, too. Please visit www.TheBaldieMovement.org to learn more and to show your support.

We also encourage you to visit www.NAAF.org to learn more about the National Alopecia Aerata Foundation. THIS non-profit is the recipient of our annual weekend retreat and beauty bazaar. Join us in Daytona Beach on the 3rd weekend in September for the Bold Beautiful & Bald Beauty Bazaar!

Thank you to "Da Bee Hive Intern Crew" at Angie BEE Productions. I would also like to thank my family for assisting me with the completion of this project; especially my beloved husband Bartee. Not only did he assist with me narration and sponsor commercial production, but he loves me unconditionally with, or without hair. Thank you, Bartee!

These stories shall continue!

Follow Confinement Chronicles By Angie BEE productions on Facebook and visit www.ConfinementChronicles.com

Be safe and BEE Blessed

Sincerely,

Evangelist Angie BEE

THE AUTHORS
In Order of Appearance

Michelle Walters-Johnson, is the owner of Lady Behind the Wig and the Luxe Hair by Michelle wig line. She's a daughter, a sister, a mother, a wife and a loyal friend. She has a Bachelor's degree in Psychology and a Master's in Business Administration. When she is not slaying wigs or giving advice, she works as an admission counselor helping people accomplish their graduate school dreams.

She suffered from hair loss. Losing her hair caused her to have to seek solutions to camouflage her hair loss, which eventually led her to the world of wigs, which then led her to wanting to share her craft with others.

By coming forward with her truth, she believes that she has found her profound purpose and unique ministry.

In the hair business self-esteem is a primary focus. Women especially, base their self-esteem on their appearance. Losing one's hair is devastating for most people. Michelle focuses on helping women with hair loss feel better about themselves. She influences them to embrace their natural beauty, and help them to realize that they have different hair replacement options available to them. If anyone suffering from hair loss is looking for support, a listening ear, a shoulder to (virtually) cry on, she is here. Please reach out to her via social media @ladybehindthewig or visit her website at www.ladybehindthewig.com

Lorna Mastin While many may feel that they need more money, more time or more resources to make their dreams come true, she knows firsthand that without a mindset shift, those things won't matter. As a coach, mentor and doula to women of all ages, Lorna Mastin is best known for guiding women through changing their mind—ushering them from a place of poverty, to personal purpose and prosperity. Where others often see destitution and desperation, Lorna has mastered bringing out the best in others. Her strategic gift for uncovering and growing other people's gifts, talents and visions continues to open doors for her in both public and private sectors—further positioning her as an expert amongst the competition. Unlike other leaders, who are often taught or trained to lead over time, it was evident early on in life that she was a natural born leader. Her innate ability to solve problems, offer wisdom and insight beyond her years, and pull greatness out of others that they didn't see within themselves didn't just make her a success at Big Brothers, Big Sisters. It set her up for success in life in general. For

Lorna, "Where there's a will, there's a way" isn't just a catchy slogan. It's a lifestyle. After overcoming low self-esteem and suicidal thoughts, she learned the true power of the mind and the mouth, igniting the passion within to redefine the mind of women worldwide. That passion unlocked unlimited opportunities for growth and expansion in both her personal and professional life. She is a mentor for the National Alopecia Areata Foundation. In addition to serving as program director for the Daughters of Citadel mentoring group, Lorna also served as YASC president and advisor for years. As a former strategic coordinator intern for NLC Consultants, she also planned and hosted events for celebrities and professional athletes. Holding both a certification in Massage Therapy and Life Coaching. She earned a Bachelor of Kinesiology, and obtained her Master's degree in Sports Administration. Through her nonprofit organization, Priceless Rubies, she encourages and empowers women to be the best version of themselves—in business, family, finances and relationships. Whether she's hosting a fitness fun event, comedy show fundraiser, her Annual Project Redefined, or giving back to the community, she has the drive and tenacity to simply get things done where others see impossibility. Offering workshops and programs that equip attendees with the necessary tools for success, her extensive arsenal of resources and connections makes winning easy for even the beginning entrepreneur or budding student. For more information or booking, visit www.pricelessrubies.com or email pricelessrubies88@gmail.com

Shay Bolling is a thirty-three-year old hairstylist & entrepreneur in Sacramento, California. She currently does hair and has a vision to launch her own hairline in January 2021, with the bigger vision of making wigs for women who suffer from hair loss, be if from cancer, alopecia, or any kind of hair loss. She would like to eventually be able to give back to her city and around the world to teenage girls who can't afford quality hair services. "My vision is indeed bigger than me!" Shay decided to be a hairstylist because she loved having the ability of connecting with women from many different walks of life and making them feel beautiful through the power of hair. Contact Shay by sending an email to southernbaby2009@gmail.com.

Uniqua Sade Leak was born May 6, 1991, in Detroit Michigan. She graduated from Consortium College Preparatory high school in 2009. Leak certified in 2010 as a Nursing Assistant from Henry Ford Community College. By 2013 Uniqua had become a registered Medical assistant through Kaplan Career Institute. She has been commissioned to numerous nursing facilities and hospitals throughout the Metro-Detroit with pride. In the summer of 2017, Uniqua earned her Associates of Arts from Wayne County Community

College district and currently serves as a Medical Assistant Instructor and float ER Technician. The medical field is a difficult career, but Leak says "it's what I love to do". Uniqua keeps herself busy, she opened an organic body product line (UniquelyU). After having two children, Uniqua learned the importance of "knowing her rights as a women." She decided to start her own Birth and postpartum Doula company (Unique Doula Services) to serve teen moms and other women in need of a support partner. She currently attends Wayne State University and is majoring in Public health. Uniqua hopes to work in infectious disease in the near future. Uniqua is an Alopecia advocate, Warrior, and sister.

For more information: Uniqua.leak@gmail.com Facebook: Uniqua Leak, Instagram: @Sadeuniquee2 and @uniquedoulaservices

Tamara Flake is the visionary behind the brand iRockitBald. This organization began as a social media handle on Instagram in 2012. The brand took off in September of 2016, when Tamara began going live telling her alopecia story for Alopecia Awareness Month. Since then, iRockitBald has been featured in the Hats off Alopecia Fashion Shows, Bald Beautiful and Bold Fashion Show, The Keep Smiling Movement – Bald Beautiful and Bold Edition, Fear of Oxygen Documentary, Bald Life Magazine, The William Malcolm Show, multiple radio shows and speaking engagements throughout the city of Detroit.

The primary mission of iRockitBald is to uplift individuals living with hair loss due to alopecia at whatever point in their journey they may be. It is the mission of iRockitBald to encourage those living with alopecia to embrace their truth, build strength and courage through loving yourself. To support you through the transition and process of Rocking It Bald or not. The primary focus is building self-love and confidence.

The vision of iRockitBald is to educate, encourage, motivate and uplift individuals living with or loving someone with hair loss. We desire to connect individuals to medical professionals and resources i.e., dermatologist, endocrinologists, psychologists through online platforms and by hosting meet and greets, community awareness events, seminars, webinars, fundraisers, walks, parties, fashion shows, trips, conferences, and virtual events.

If you are someone struggling with an alopecia diagnosis or hair loss, we recommend you take some time to self-assess and identify what you love about you. Self-love is the number one key. Then surround yourself with people who care for you unconditionally and support your truth.

Surround yourself with likeminded individuals; seek them out socially at in person events or via social media. Educate yourself, know your worth and do what makes you feel your best. Most importantly, it is your process. Take as long as you need to grow through it. For more information or booking please visit www.irockitbald.com or email irockitbald@gmail.com.

Raquel Johnson is fifty years old born in Benton Harbor, Michigan, and raised in Detroit. She has one son who is thirty-three and one grandson who is twelve. She has been employed by Blue Cross Blue Shield of Michigan for twenty-two years, and she is currently a senior analyst. She has Bachelors in Business Leadership and Masters in Health Care Administration.

You may contact her at Rdennis88@yahoo.com. Her favorite scripture is Romans 8:38-39.

Bartee is affectionately referred to as "The Rage of The Stage" here in Central Florida. This sensational R&B singer began his career at the age of eleven in his hometown of Akron, Ohio. He continues to share his natural-born feeling for music just as aggressively as he first did decades ago. Always sought after, Bartee is a versatile entertainer that performs Smooth Jazz, Vintage Soul, and a beautiful Motown Review.

Bartee has shared the stage with music icons such as James Ingram, Howard Hewitt, The Ohio Players, Linda Cole, and The O'Jays. Bartee leads the Dads-on-Duty workshop while on *The TOUR that Angie BEE Presents*, and he leads by Angie BEE's side in the God, Me & You Workshop, as well. You can find Bartee performing a Motown Review concert during the TOUR weekend retreats for couples, and he continues to serve the Lord with gladness through his lifestyle and commitment to his family.

In 2013, Bartee met, dated, and married Angie BEE in less than six months. Before he met her, he vowed to NEVER remarry, and she vowed NEVER to submit to another man. God orchestrated something different for the two of them, and their book reveals the details.

Bartee first became a published author on August 1, 2017. As co-author, he and his wife Angie BEE wrote *In the Beginning: There Was God, Me & You*, published by Ladero Press. This book reveals their true love story that only God could have written. Bartee always wanted to write a book and he will soon write his life story of juvenile incarceration to prison, and God's many blessings in his life.

Together, Bartee and Angie BEE have two sons, two daughters and two brand new sons-in-law.

Follow him at: www.BarteeSings.com and www.facebook.com/pg/BarteeTheAuthor.

You know, my husband may joke around a bit about my round, bald head, but he is truthful about ONE thing...most men (people) can recognize a person wearing a wig from a mile away! Why do we wear them? Are we trying to impress somebody else or do we cover our heads in shame? Either way, I appreciate my husband's jovial nature about my bald head. Even though he is bald-by-choice, I appreciate HIS bald head, too!

Angie BEE's hairdresser was the first to find a bald spot in the crown of her head, at the age of 28. By the time she was 30, Angie BEE was diagnosed with Alopecia Areata after receiving the results of a biopsy. She dealt with the embarrassment and the shame by constantly wearing a wig.

Ordained as an Evangelist in 2014, Angie BEE entered menopause. 'The hot flashes were horrible. I snatched off that wig every chance I got!" she shared.

Encouraged by her husband Bartee, Angie BEE finally gathered the courage to go on a dinner date with her husband, without wearing her wig. The servers at the restaurant showered her with compliments, and her confidence grew!

By 2016, Angie BEE & Bartee were encouraged by community advocate Donna Gray-Banks to have an event to encourage and teach others with Alopecia. In 2017, the very first Bold Beautiful & Bald Beauty Bazaar for Alopecia Awareness took place in Daytona Beach, Florida. A donation from the proceeds was donated to the National Alopecia Areata Foundation at www.NAAF.org

Since that inaugural event, attendees have arrived from Michigan, Ohio, North Carolina, Texas, and multiple cities throughout Florida. Each attendee learned about various forms of Alopecia, wig options, and how to use a head covering along with makeup and eyelash application.

Followers joined the group page at www.BoldBeautifulAndBald.com Weekend retreat attendees continued to participate despite the pandemic and fashion show cancellation in 2020. Men, women, and children attended.

Angie BEE and her husband Bartee are participating members of the Central Florida Alopecia Support Group in Eatonville, Florida. They organized support group outings in Volusia County prior to the pandemic and they presented Alopecia Awareness fashion show events in Detroit and Atlanta.

As the "slap seen and heard around the world" Oscar controversy emerged, Angie BEE was interviewed and featured in a two-page cover story in the Daytona Times Newspaper. As she shared her Alopecia journey in the news story, she invited families to attend the 6th annual beauty bazaar and announced the debut of the new website at www.BoldBeautifulAndBald.com

www.ingramcontent.com/pod-product-compliance
Lightning Source LLC
Chambersburg PA
CBHW070028030426
42335CB00017B/2335